What Others are Saying about *Women of Strength*:

"When I picked up this book, I had no idea what I was in for. The author's introduction felt like a page from my own personal diary. This book seems to be just what I needed to get my battle with the bulge back on track. The way the author relates our spiritual life with our physical life is eye-opening. This book is short, but each day's "devotion" is worth savoring. I will be checking out more of these books, for sure!" ~ Pauline C.

"I had backslidden on my exercising and had been depressed about it for a few months, so I started reading this book expecting to feel guilty and disillusioned about my lack of commitment to something I know is so important. But instead I was encouraged. Ms. Payne gives practical advice on how to get back on track and overcome some of the obstacles that get in the way of all of us - like lack of time, setting realistic goals, and developing a plan of action. I am encouraged to get back on track. Now I realize, by starting and not condemning myself (which is really more painful), I can work toward being a woman of strength and even enjoy the process!"~ Lorilyn R.

"I really like how the author laid out this book. It's different and creative. The sections are divided into seasons instead of days/weeks. Also, she does a great job combining health tips with spiritual growth. I like how each section has work-out questions she answers and has an actual work-out/exercise you can do. I recommend this to anyone who wants to get inspired to take care of their body and spirit." ~ Krystal K.

"This book would be great for personal use. I can also see it being a good resource for a woman's Bible study group in the way it brings up a variety of topics for discussion, deals with seasonal challenges, encourages healthy living, and has a built-in activity (exercise) component. You'll make fit ladies out of us all yet, Kim!" ~ Violet N.

"This unique, practical, inspirational book reflects the author's quest to help other women improve their spiritual and physical health through the seasons. Get your copy and get healthy, physically and spiritually. I give it a 5-star rating!" ~ Carol R.

"I would DEFINITELY recommend this book as a devotional for women who are trying to keep their bodies (God's temple), minds, and spirits, healthy." ~ Penny H.

"I really enjoyed this devotional. It is different than any other devotional I currently have and enjoyed the change. Just reading this devotional inspired me to be more physically active and exercise as well as spend more time with God. Recommended! " ~ Shelley H.

"As I was reading this book I noticed that actually became calm and very encouraged instead of shamed and useless...It does not give you an overwhelming "MUST DO" push but a loving, gentle and even funny way to get healthy. And the added bonus and most important by using God's Word intertwined all throughout. Kimberley, yet again another book you have written that I truly recommend to any woman!!!!!!!" ~ Karen L.

Women of Strength – a devotional to improve spiritual and physical health

Copyright 2015 Kimberley Payne

All inquiries should be addressed to: www.kimberleypayne.com

Caution:
This program provides a general overview on this topic and may not apply to everyone. The information contained in this book is intended to be solely informational and educational. In view of the complex, individual, and specific nature of health and fitness problems, this book is not intended to replace professional medical advice. It is assumed the *Women of Strength* participant will consult a medical or health professional before beginning this or any other weight-loss or physical fitness program. The author expressly disclaims any responsibility for any liability, loss, or risk, personal or otherwise, which is incurred as a consequence, directly or indirectly, of the use and application of any of the contents of this book.

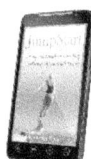 **Your Free Gift**

JumpStart – Launch your journey to improve physical and spiritual fitness

Want to make simple changes to improve spiritual and physical health? Discover a daily, specific program to create a routine.

Visit https://www.kimberleypayne.com/jumpstart/

Table of Contents

Introduction

I created this devotional book out of a desire to become more physically healthy. As a former personal trainer, I knew all about exercise and nutrition, however, I still missed something. Or should I say, Someone.

In the past, I'd never included God in my health and fitness plan. I thought it wasn't something worthy of His attention. However, God checked my spirit and told me that He wants to be part of everything in my life; even something as small as losing a few pounds.

How can you become a woman of strength today?

You can honour your body by taking care of it–both physically and spiritually. *Women of Strength* is the perfect companion for your health program. There are four divisions to follow the seasons – winter, spring, summer, autumn. Each season is further divided into 6 sections that include an inspirational devotional, a fact on common health and fitness questions, a reflection, a prayer, a Bible verse, and an energizing exercise.

My prayer is for you to improve your spiritual and physical health through the seasons!

Kimberley Payne

God is in the details

I gained a pound in the last week. It really is remarkable how a small number on the scale can have such great significance. Last week, I didn't gorge and eat with gluttonous hunger. I didn't sit down to seven-course meals and midnight snacks. No, the error I made wasn't in the big sense but rather in the small. I neglected to mind what I ate. That is, I didn't pay attention. I ignored my body signals of hunger and fullness. I ate food while tending to other matters – as if eating were second to other activities. I ate food for the mere taste of it and, more often than not, I ate without fully knowing I was eating.

When I am mindful of what I eat I truly enjoy it. I look to it as a source of pleasure and nourishment. When I treat food with respect I treat my body with respect. It is the same with my Christian behaviour. Some days, I tend to get lazy with my worship of God and just go through the motions. I may go to church but my mind is tending to other matters. When I'm not mindful of my prayers and pay lip service to them, they come only from my mind but not my heart. It's not enough to practice spiritual rituals. I must worship God with my heart as well as my mouth.

My intentions may be good but if I don't pay enough attention to the Word, I realize that I haven't lived up to my true call as a Christian. Although I didn't commit a horrendous sin, my behaviour isn't reflected in the large events. Instead, it's the small details. Was I patient and slow to anger? Did I respect the clerk behind the counter, obviously overwhelmed by the volume of customers? Was I kind and gentle with my children? I realize that my misbehaviour hurts God more than anyone else.

I pray that I won't be like those spoken of in Isaiah 29:13, "The Lord says: These people come near to me with their mouth and honor me with their lips, but their hearts are far from me. Their worship of me is made up only of rules taught by men."

I don't want to go through the motions, but rather, I want to pay attention to the details of my heart. God is in the little things. He is in the every day. If I look to Him in my everyday life, I'll grow spiritually strong. I want to be healthy in body, mind and spirit.

Exercise Your Funny Bone

The Best Vitamin for a Christian: B1

You Asked

Q: Do I need to spend hours in the gym to see results from an exercise program?

A: Even if you don't have time for a formal workout during your day, any exercise is better than none. Try to take three 10-minute walks. For strength training, three 20-minute sessions a week will do the job.

Faith Lift

Dear Father – I pray that You will provide me with the courage to accept Your power and make the changes You ask of me. In Jesus' name, I pray.

Reflection

Yesterday, I spent the majority of my time outdoors playing in the snow. I got some good cardio activity from clearing the front walkway and back deck. Then I built a snow fort to play war with my son and his best friend. And, if I may say so myself, the fort looked fantastic!

What are you doing to enjoy the season your in now?

Top Tip

Check with your doctor – You should get medical clearance from your physician before making any significant changes in your physical activity level.

Bible Truth

"Don't you know that you yourselves are God's temple and that God's Spirit lives in you" (1 Corinthians 3:16 NIV)?

Challenge

Drink one less caffeine beverage every day.

Praise Move: Legs - Lunge

Stand holding a dumbbell in each hand, your hands next to your thighs and palms facing your body.

Keep your feet hip-width apart, knees slightly bent, abdominals contracted.

Take a long stride forward so that your knee is directly over your heel and your thigh is almost parallel to the floor.

Your rear leg should be relaxed and bent so that the knee almost touches the floor.

Hold this position for a moment, and then push back to the starting position. Repeat 10 times.

Repeat for other leg.

<u>Tips</u>

1. The forward flexed knee should not extend past the forward foot.
2. Keep your upper body in line with your hips.
3. Learn proper technique before adding weight.

Resolutions

I did it all wrong. During the Christmas season, I stopped doing the things that I needed to do in order to be right with me, and to be right with the world, but most importantly to be right with God.

My first error happened by choosing to go to bed much later than normal. Over the Christmas holidays, I would allow the children to stay up later than their regular bedtime, and then found myself eventually going to bed a few hours later. I threw off my body clock.

I made my second mistake by allowing my body to dictate when I felt like getting up. I know from years of experience that the process of waking up – no matter what time it is – is slow and painful for me. I will feel as groggy and resentful about being yanked from my warm, cozy bed after a six-hour sleep as I would after a twelve-hour slumber. So, when I relied on my body to signal me to wake I would actually stay in bed extra hours then feel guilty for sleeping in. These two mistakes threw my physical and emotional state into alarm because I changed my routine.

Then to further upset my system, I stopped taking my morning walk. Usually after I walked the children to the bus stop, I would continue on for another forty-five minutes. This provided a time to get my body moving, my blood flowing and my mind thinking. Without this walk, I didn't get my usual energy surge needed for the day. Without this morning boost, I felt like I needed to drag myself everywhere. I also didn't have the enthusiasm or desire to do my other exercise – strength training. I went into a downward spiral.

Physically and emotionally, I suffered. Add to this the new chores and unique assignments of the holiday season. I shopped when I normally would be reading. I wrapped when I normally would be writing. In addition to this, I cooked, cleaned and prepared for festivities.

As if that were not enough, I had two children home from school for two weeks. I love my children – let's get that straight from the start – but they are kids. They bicker and argue and they complain and fight. And they love me. They want to spend time with Mom. They want to help Mom shop, wrap and cook (they never want to clean though). They want Mom to play with them, to read to them, to be with them.

Too much sleep, no exercise and children all day -- they were the ingredients for a stressful holiday season.

However, I had neglected one other thing that could have truly helped me. I didn't spend time with God. Oh, I continued to pray at meals and bedtime. However, I didn't spend quality, one-on-one, reflective time with Him.

On my morning walks, I would do more than look at the passing homes. I practice my walking meditation. It's a time when I connect with God and talk to Him through my thoughts and prayers. It's a mindful and special time between us that I have come to cherish. On my walks, I explore my life and give praise and thanksgiving for what He has given me. I open my heart and pour out my troubles. I give thought to others and pray for the needs of my family, friends and community. Without my morning walk, I had not only missed out on the healthy physical benefits, but more importantly, I'd denied the spiritual healing it had provided.

Generally after my morning walk, I return home to hot coffee and my pen and paper. I spend one hour writing. I record any enlightenment God has shown me and I reflect on the prayers I had offered up. It's a time for me to not only talk with God, but to listen for a response. For the entire Christmas season, I had not done this. Not once!

Lastly, I didn't spend time in His Word. My usual routine affords me time each day to spend reading and studying the Bible. But because the time set aside wasn't given its usual priority, it became lost.

I enjoyed my holidays. No one suffered illness this year and we had opportunity to visit many relatives. However, each day took a little bit more out of me and by the end of the month, I felt very drained.

God is the only thing that really rejuvenates me. He feeds me each day. He gives me the energy and enthusiasm needed to get through the day.

I'll take this past Christmas season as a lesson for my life. My resolution is to pledge my life anew to Jesus. Although routines change, and life can throw me curves, I resolve to spend quality time with God first and foremost every single day in order to be right with me, to be right with the world, and most importantly to be right with God.

"Therefore, if anyone is in Christ, he is a new creation; the old has gone, the new has come" (2 Corinthians 5:17 NIV)!

Exercise Your Funny Bone

Seven days without prayer makes one weak.

You Asked

Q: I heard that low-intensity exercise wouldn't promote weight loss like high intensity exercise. Is this true?

A: The most important factor for losing body fat is the total calories burned, regardless of the rate at which they are burned. The benefit of working out at a lower intensity is that you won't get as tired as quickly.

Faith Lift

Dear Lord – I pray that You will help me to stop trying to prove I am good enough. In Jesus' name, I pray.

Reflection

The days seem short when the sun rises much later and sets much earlier. I ventured out in the evening again to take the dog for a walk around the block with my husband and daughter. Upon our return from around the circle, my 8-year-old son and his best friend bombarded us. They had been waiting to ambush us from their snow forts. We took the challenge, and with Jessie, the dog, on our side, we were able to push them into a retreat. It exhilarated me! If you haven't tried a snowball fight lately, I would highly recommend it.

What fun activity have you tried lately?

Top Tip

Take it slow and steady – Remember that fitness is not a "quick fix". This is a lifestyle change and you may experience setbacks and plateaus. Think of this program as a start to a whole new lifestyle.

Bible Truth

"No temptation has seized you except what is common to man. And God is faithful; he will not let you be tempted beyond what you can bear. But when you are tempted, he will also provide a way out so that you can stand up under it" (1 Corinthians 10:13 NIV).

Challenge

Go through your closet and give away or throw away any clothes that you haven't worn in the last two years. When you buy something new – give away something else.

Praise Move: Legs - Standing Side Leg Lift

Stand with your feet hip-width apart.

With an ankle weight securely around your ankle, face a wall or the back of a chair and hold it with both hands for support.

Lift one leg outward and upward to the side only as high as you can while maintaining torso and hip position.

Lower leg slowly and return to starting position. Repeat 10 times.

Repeat for other leg.

Tips:

1. Contract your abdominals so your tailbone is pointing to the floor.
2. If you feel any back discomfort, don't lift your leg so high.
3. Keep your knee slightly bent.

Habits

A friend asked how she could apply a calm, meditative state of mind in her otherwise busy agitated life. How could she become a centered, joyful person when she is in the full force of daily living?

I don't have all the answers, however, I could offer her some ideas of what works for me. My first suggestion was to spend time with God. Easy enough, however, the old argument starts, "The problem is just that – I don't have time! How can you ask me to add something to my to-do-list? I don't have enough time."

I feel that time is not the real problem. It is the perceived problem. It is created in the mind and this is where the problem originates. The mind is where that infernal tape keeps repeating, "You don't have time. You'll never get that done. Look how much you have to do. You don't have time. You'll never get that done. Look how much you have to do. You don't have time…" And it repeats continually.

Spending time with God settles this voice and eventually it'll be a mere whisper and finally it'll be gone. The important thing is to seek God every day. Not on a superficial level or a theoretical level but it's to connect with Him on a spiritual level. It's to get in the routine of being with Him. I've developed some habits that help me to do this:

Create a quiet space

This is a place where I can go to be refreshed with no television and no telephone. I brew some hot tea, light a scented candle and play relaxing music. Then I sit quietly. I do this everyday. My body is conditioned to relax in response to these stimuli.

Read

What we feed our minds affects our body and our spirit. The Bible is an obvious choice and I like to read one chapter of Proverbs and pick one specific proverb that speaks to me that day. There are also excellent Christian books and magazines including Bible-in-a-year books, devotionals, Oswald Chambers, and many on-line resources.

Walk

This gets me out to enjoy the beauty of the world around me, not just the four walls of my home. On this walk, I tune into my five senses recognizing all that I see, smell, taste, feel and hear. Then I pray. I open with praise to God and thank Him for the good in my life. Then I continue on my walk in prayer for others. This takes away the self-centeredness that can become like a destructive tonic. Thinking of others and praying for them is an effective way to stay healthy and focused. The walk need not be more than ten minutes to feel physically challenged and emotionally released.

Write

In my writing, I purposely identify five new things every day for which I'm grateful. This has an amazing impact on my attitude and really helps put things into perspective. It helps to take a step back and see the big picture and not get so entangled in the nitty-gritty details of the day.

Other Ideas

Other people meditate. Still others listen and dance to music. Use whatever suits your personality as long as it's the same each day and your body, mind and spirit connect and you are able to communicate with God. This may be difficult for some – shift workers, moms with little ones – but just being able to take five minutes should be enough. Every minute spent with God will help you to be more calm, centered and joyful.

"Be joyful always; pray continually; give thanks in all circumstances, for this is God's will for you in Christ Jesus" (1 Thessalonians 5:16-18 NIV).

Exercise Your Funny Bone

Prayer - Wireless access to God with no roaming charges

You Asked

Q: I only have time for a 30-minute workout. Is stretching important?

A: Yes it is. Strength and endurance exercises tend to shorten muscles and therefore reduce elasticity. In order to improve flexibility, these exercises must be combined with slow, gently stretching exercises.

Faith Lift

Dear Lord – I pray that You will remind me each day that You are at work within me and around me. In Jesus' name, I pray.

Reflection

Winter can be fun. I had a great game of baseball with my son. It started rather innocently; while I shoveled the front walkway my 8-year old winged me with a snowball. I quickly lifted the shovel and caught the ball in the air with a perfect hit. It sprayed everywhere! My son thought this a delight and so continued to fire ball after ball at me. I must say that I batted great; the head of the shovel is much better than any aluminum bat.

What fun sport or game can you make up?

Top Tip

Schedule exercise in – Take an honest look at how you spend your days. Schedule exercise in your daily planner just as you would with a business meeting or a doctor's appointment.

Bible Truth

"And the God of all grace, who called you to his eternal glory in Christ, after you have suffered a little while, will Himself restore you and make you strong, firm and steadfast" (1 Peter 5:10 NIV).

Challenge

Don't watch television for at least one day per week for a month. You would be amazed how much time has been freed up. Television is a ferocious time waster.

Praise Move: Legs - Wall Slide

Stand with your back to a wall, feet parallel to each other.

Keep your back straight against the wall.

Bend your knees to slide slowly down the wall.

Your lower legs should remain parallel to the wall.

Hold this position for 8 counts, then slide slowly up the wall. Repeat 10 times.

Tips:

1. Don't lean into the wall; use it for balance only.
2. Don't let your thighs go any lower than parallel to the floor.
3. Contract your abdominals throughout the move.

Just Do It

It looked like a gorgeous day outside. Fresh snow covered the landscape and trees were heavy with a blanket of white. The sun reflected off the field in a splash of sparkles – it appeared to be another beautiful winter day. But the thermometer stood at minus 20 in the sunshine. I cancelled my walk (yet again) because of the cold.

For months, my routine was to get my children ready in the morning, walk them to the bus stop and then walk around the neighbourhood by myself. However, my routine became interrupted when I started a new work schedule and so instead of walking to the bus stop I drove the children. Then other days in the week seemed to become busier and I found myself itching to get to my office to clear away the things of the day. Instead of starting my day with a walk around the block, I started to weigh it up against other conflicting priorities. Now, the act of walking had to convince me of its worth. Each day a battle raged – walk or not walk?

What I learned is that when I didn't give myself the choice, I went for a walk regardless of temperature or mood. However, when I made walking an option, I had to think each day, "Am I up to it? Do I have time for it? Is it warm enough or cool enough or dry enough?" Each day I put myself through a dance of questions, instead of just doing it. "Just do it" (the saying made famous by Nike) has tremendous impact. If I would walk in the morning, instead of giving myself the option, I wouldn't have to worry about what's more important on my list of things to do. I would return from my walk refreshed and ready to face the day.

This reminds me of time spent in prayer and Bible study. When I make it a regular part of my routine then there is no question that I'll do it. For months, I had dedicated thirty minutes from 4:00-4:30 p.m. to quiet time with God. The kids were home from school; I reviewed their homework and fed them a snack. Then while they had free time to play – before chores, supper and evening extracurricular activities – I'd steal away to read my Bible. The kids knew that this was, "Mommy's time with God." And they left me alone for thirty minutes. However, now my job requires that on some days I'm not home until after 4:30. My routine has changed. On days that I am home I'm no longer disciplined to take the time in prayer. Instead, I wonder about what to make for supper. I tidy up the house and finish up details on the computer. My quiet time with God is now competing against my to-do list. Whereas before I would "just do it" now each day becomes a battle of what I feel is more important at the moment.

My lesson? Just do it! I need to plan out my week in advance knowing my work schedule and my "to do" list; make contingencies for those days that my regular walking and devotion time gets interrupted, and then do it without further thought.

Exercise Your Funny Bone

When down in the mouth, remember Jonah. He came out all right.

You Asked

Q: My heart rate is 50 bpm. Is it better to have a higher resting heart rate?

A: A normal resting heart rate can vary from as low as 40 beats per minute (bpm) to as high as 100 bpm, with an average of 75 bpm for women. Physical activity helps the heart muscle to pump more efficiently for an optimal resting heart rate.

Faith Lift

Dear God – I pray that You will help me to see myself as You do, to see my own worth and respect myself. In Jesus' name, I pray.

Reflection

Recently, I tried some interval training. I walked for a bit, then jogged for a bit. I did this the whole way of my regular walk for 45-minutes. My heart and lungs handled it well. But I felt as if I weighed 800 pounds -- my calves were on fire, my hips ached, my upper body itched from the bouncing. When I told a friend, she encouraged me to continue practicing and said that it'll only get better. I'll take her word for it and continue with my new routine.

What new activity would you consider trying?

Top Tip

Create space – Create an area to call your own and make exercise so accessible that you have no excuse. Buy some low-priced equipment: an exercise bike, a resistance band, a set of dumbbells, a stretching mat, a jump rope and an exercise video.

Bible Truth

"The bolts of your gates will be iron and bronze, and your strength will equal your days" (Deuteronomy 33:25 NIV).

Challenge

Try a new routine, a new exercise, and/or a new time of the day to exercise.

Praise Move: Shoulder - Side Raise

Stand holding a dumbbell in each hand, arms by your sides, palms facing side leg. Lead with bent elbows and slowly raise the weight out to your sides to shoulder height without rotating the arms.

Your palms should face the floor at the top position with arms parallel to the floor.

Pause briefly at the top of the move, than slowly lower the weights to the starting position.

Repeat 10 times.

Tips:

1. Keep your arms straight without locking your elbows.
2. Avoid swinging the arms up using momentum to lift the weight.
3. Keep your neck relaxed and your shoulders stationary.

The Body

As a former personal fitness trainer, I've learned that there are many parts to our body. I studied kinesiology. I learned about our muscles, bones, tendons and ligaments. I trained to see how one affects the other and how to exercise them properly.

As a Christian, I've learned that there are many parts to the Body of Christ. When we talk about the Body, we are talking about all Christians.

"It was He who gave some to be apostles, some to be prophets, some to be evangelists, and some to be pastors and teachers, to prepare God's people for works of service, so that the Body of Christ may be built up" (Ephesians 4:11-12 NIV).

Each one of us is different and the Body of Christ is not made up of one part, but of many. And like our physical body, the Body of Christ is dependent on each part to work properly in order for the whole to function.

Without eyes, the physical body cannot see. Without hands, it cannot touch. Without ears, it cannot hear. The Body of Christ is the same. God uses pastors to pastor His flock. God heals through healers. He uses prophets to prophesy.

Each part works toward the betterment of the whole. We are the Body of Christ, and each one of us is a part of it.

"And in the church God has appointed first of all apostles, second prophets, third teachers, then workers of miracles, also those having gifts of healing, those able to help others, those with gifts of administration, and those speaking in different kinds of tongues" (1 Corinthians 12:28 NIV).

It is important that we know and understand how we fit within the Body of Christ. Some people work well behind the scenes to ensure details are looked after. Some people work best ministering to others through music and song. Some people are gifted with teaching children about the Bible. What we need to do is find out our role in the Body of Christ and use it to the full glory of God.

It's not complicated to find out your role in the Body, but it does take time. There are many wonderful resources including programs and books on the internet.

Exercise Your Funny Bone

If you want the last word, apologize.

You Asked

Q: When I stop weight training, does muscle change to fat?

A: Muscle and fat are two different types of tissue; you can't turn one into another. The bulk of your fat sits right under your skin, on top of your muscle. You can increase your muscle mass, and you can decrease body fat, but one doesn't directly affect the other. When you stop strength training your muscles will shrink somewhat. If you don't decrease your food intake when you stop training, the extra calories that you'd normally have burned up in activity will turn into fat.

Faith Lift

Dear God – When I turn to You I pray that I will feel a quieting down and my energy will be replenished. In Jesus' name, I pray.

Reflection

Building a healthy body is similar to building a house. To build a house, a general contractor and specific trade's people are hired. A bricklayer is as important as a plumber for a complete house. Just the same, building a body requires all the components of health; cardiovascular exercise, strength training, flexibility and nutrition. I can't ignore any aspect and expect to have a solid foundation of wellness

What component of health have you been neglecting?

Top Tip

Track your progress – Keep a chart of your progress and small improvements will become noticeable. Track your sets, repetitions and weight on a program card.

Bible Truth

"For everything God created is good" (1 Timothy 4:4 NIV).

Challenge

Set a goal. The goal must be SMART - Specific, Measurable, Attainable, Realistic and Time-oriented.

Praise Move: Chest - Bench Press

Lie face up on a flat bench with your feet on the floor.

Hold a barbell over your mid-chest with an overhand grip a little wider than shoulder-width apart, arms straight but not locked.

Slowly lower the barbell toward your chest until it almost touches.

At the bottom, your forearms and wrists are perpendicular to the floor and parallel with each other.

Press the barbell up to the starting position. Repeat 10 times.

<u>Tips</u>:

1. If your feet don't reach the floor, put them on the bench.
2. Don't bounce the barbell off your chest.
3. Rely on muscle, not momentum, to push bar back to starting position.

Faithfulness

I find myself back in the place I sat two short years ago – waiting. I remember the uncomfortable wait and the questions that surrounded it. When will our home sell? When will we move? When will we find a new home? It felt like a free fall. I had no idea where I would be living or what I would be doing. For a chronic list maker and goal planner the unknowns were extremely disturbing.

I remember the stress affected me emotionally, spiritually and most obviously, physically. I gained quite a bit of weight and my face broke out in pimples. I had little energy to face the day and lacked motivation because of my lack of direction.

I felt as if I stood in the desert. Looking back, I see that it was the calm before the storm – time that I should have spent in preparation instead of anxiety. I could have used that downtime to finish projects that I've always wanted to do (like put photos in albums) instead of spending my energies asking questions and worrying. But it's said that hindsight is 20/20. How come I find it so hard to learn from experience?

I believe that any day now questions will be answered, lists will be full of things to do and I will again plan out my goals. I need to look back at my past experiences and see how God has been faithful. I need to remember all the times where I felt like I stood in the desert, only to find an oasis some time later.

We need to learn from past experiences by keeping them in our memory. When we look back at God's faithfulness in the past we can find peace knowing He will take care of us in the future.

One way to keep a constant reminder of God's faithfulness is through a Prayer Journal. Every time we have a prayer, it can be entered into the journal leaving a space open to record the date God answered.

Looking back, I see that God answered my prayer. We sold our home for more than we expected to get. We bought a home closer to family than we imagined, with all of the comforts we wanted. Learning from past experiences to remember God's faithfulness can be made a little easier when we use a Prayer Journal. Why not start one today?

"Know therefore that the Lord your God is God; he is the faithful God, keeping His covenant of love to a thousand generations of those who love Him and keep His commands" (Deuteronomy 7:9 NIV).

Exercise Your Funny Bone

God answers knee-mail.

You Asked

Q: To "warm up" do I just need to stretch a muscle?

A: No, to warm up muscles, begin with gentle movement from activities that create a slight increase in blood flow and heart rate. Stretching a muscle doesn't warm it. In fact, trying to stretch a cold muscle can lead to injury and is dangerous since muscles have less elasticity when cold. First, warm up with a cardiovascular activity such as walking, and then stretch.

Faith Lift

Dear Lord – I pray that I will receive my strength through You to cope with whatever I must face each day. In Jesus' name, I pray.

Reflection

Some days it can be discouraging to look in the mirror and feel that my goal seems so far away. It's too easy to become apathetic and give up. However, I've found that paying attention to the small things – like a pair of pants that fit a little looser – is helpful to stay on track. God doesn't want me to become discouraged and give up.

What small changes have you noticed since beginning this program?

Top Tip

Follow the 10-minute rule – Decide to do only 10 minutes of exercise and then you can stop if you want. Generally, once you have started exercising you won't want to stop. If you don't have time for a full workout each day, break down your workouts into three or four smaller chunks of 10 minutes each. And you can do different things in each of these times.

Bible Truth

"But the Lord is faithful, and He will strengthen and protect you from the evil one" (2 Thessalonians 3:3 NIV).

Challenge

Write a list of thirty things that you are grateful for.

Praise Move: Chest - Push Up

Lie on your stomach, legs together. Place hands under your shoulders, fingers pointing forward.

Push up from the floor by straightening your elbows, without locking them and keep the upper body in a straight line, using the knees like a hinge.

Pause momentarily and slowly lower your chest to the starting position. Repeat 10 times.

Tips:

1. If this exercise is too difficult, begin by doing a push-up while standing and facing a wall.
2. Don't let your lower back arch or your buttocks stick up.
3. Keep your elbows close to your sides and your body in a straight line.

Temptation

I began smoking at age fifteen. I had continued the habit for over ten years before I decided to quit when I became pregnant with my first-born. Not a difficult choice – I wanted to be as healthy as possible for my child. However, it was difficult to follow through on this decision.

The habit became ingrained; I smoked on the way to work, on my breaks, lunchtime and on my drive home again. Many of my friends and co-workers also smoked. My lifestyle revolved around this habit.

The decision to quit had to involve changes. I had to change my habits – I took walks on my break and at lunchtime and chewed on a sucker on my drives. I no longer joined friends for a coffee and a cigarette. I ate sunflower seeds when the cravings became intense.

I resolved to quit for the health of my baby and myself. With my new habits in place I felt confident. However, shortly after my decision a friend reminded me of tickets I had purchased to go to a concert with six other friends. We had bought them months in advance and my excitement grew weekly. I thought I could handle this. At the concert, I enjoyed the whole scene including the loud music and cheering crowd. What fun – I felt delighted that I had agreed to join them. But once outside, my friends all lit up and I couldn't ignore the smell of a freshly lit cigarette. I begged a friend for a drag. She argued with me, but after a few moments of pleading she eventually handed over the cigarette and I took a long haul. I had an immediate reaction; a mixture of satisfaction, yearning for more, and complete disgust. My conflict felt painful. Although I desperately wanted a cigarette, I couldn't bear the repulsion I felt giving in to my craving. The guilt weighed heavy. I wished I had not gone to the concert. I wished I had not gone with my friends who still smoked. I wished I had not put myself into such a position of temptation.

When tempted, I lost. I thought I could handle the situation but I couldn't. I thought I had the strength to do it, but I didn't. I decided not to put myself into such a place of temptation again.

This is what it must mean in the Bible when it says to flee from temptation. Instead of thinking we can fight against it, we shouldn't even put ourselves in that position. We should run from it. First Timothy 6:11 tells us to flee from all this.

Temptation itself is not a sin. We are all exposed to temptation – even Jesus was tempted (Matthew 4:1 NIV). However, yielding to temptation is a sin. The easiest way to not yield to temptation is to resist it and run from it.

"Submit yourselves, then, to God. Resist the devil, and he will flee from you" (James 4:7 NIV).

Exercise Your Funny Bone

God so loved the world that He did not send a committee.

You Asked

Q: Is a flat stomach a realistic goal for all people?

A: A perfectly flat midsection is not a realistic goal. Even if you're very thin, your internal organs may give a slight roundness there. Abdominal exercises can tighten and strengthen your stomach, but they won't reduce the layer of fat that sits on top. To shed body fat, you must burn calories through cardiovascular and strength training exercises.

Faith Lift

Dear Lord – I pray that You will give me the courage to let You control my life and that when I need assurance I can depend on You for all my needs. In Jesus' name, I pray.

Reflection

It's wonderful to be able to get outside again and enjoy the warmer weather. Last week, I had opportunity to bike around the neighbourhood, play catch with the dog, clean up the backyard, and play baseball with the family. Activity is so much easier when it's sunny and warm.

What activities do you enjoy outdoors?

Top Tip

Do something else at the same time – You can read or listen to books on tape while riding a stationary bike. You can also watch TV, listen to music, talk to God or think about a Scripture reading. If outdoors, carry a trash bag with you and collect garbage along the road or trail.

Bible Truth

"Be strong and courageous. Do not be afraid or terrified because of them, for the Lord your God goes with you; He will never leave you nor forsake you" (Deuteronomy 31:6 NIV).

Challenge

Spend ten minutes once a week gazing at the stars.

Praise Move: Back - Shrugs

Stand holding a dumbbell in each hand, arms comfortably shoulder-width apart, palms facing front thigh.

Keep your body straight, and lift the shoulders as high as possible.

Pause at the top of the movement, than lower slowly to starting position. Repeat 10 times.

Tips:

1.The arms should remain straight as the shoulders are raised.
2.Don't hold your breath throughout the movement.
3.Lift and lower the weight slowly.

Intense Interest

Spring is in full bloom and with it comes the excitement to get outdoors and try new activities. If you've been indoors this winter, watching sports more than participating in them, be especially careful when you re-start your exercise program. A good indicator of how hard you're working is the "Talk Test".

When exercising, if you can talk continually without a break, it shows that you're not working hard enough. However, when you can say only a word or two at a time before you have to take a breath you are working too hard. For example, if you say: "the other" (breath) "day" (breath) "I went" (breath) "to" (breath) "the store"...then it is obvious that you are exercising too hard. You have winded yourself.

Wearing a heart rate monitor can help to tell if you're in the correct heart rate zone for aerobic exercise. But short of wearing a monitor, a comfortable conversation may be something like: "the other day I went" (breath) "to the store" (breath).

To increase intensity, try new activities that are fun for you. A friend shares, "It has been reinforced for me that exercise that is fun is much less exhausting. Last night I played tennis for the first time in more than ten years. Because it has been so long, I signed up for a beginner class. The hottest day of the year so far, we were pretty much constantly in motion except for some short stints when we watched the instructor demonstrate a technique. Yet after 90 minutes, I still jogged across the court to pick up the tennis balls, and I didn't feel pooped like I do after 30 minutes of swimming or an hour of walking. I think it was because I was having fun - the challenge of developing and improving a skill, of getting the ball into the correct target area (okay - of just getting the ball across the net)."

Another friend shares the joy of playing tennis, "When we went away to a resort, we played tennis with our children. I thought it would only hold their interest for a short time. But they loved it. We played for at least two hours."

Whether you play tennis, swim, mountain bike or run, the most important thing is that you enjoy it. This will help you to stay at the right level of intensity and take the chore out of getting fit.

Exercise Your Funny Bone

From a church bulletin: The ladies of the church have cast off clothing of every kind. They may be seen in the basement on Friday afternoon.

You Asked

Q: I feel that I have no time to exercise. Do I need an hour each day?

A: Exercise means active living. You can walk your dog, go for a short bicycle ride to the mailbox or take the stairs instead of an elevator. It all adds up.

Faith Lift

Dear Lord – I pray that I become what You want me to be and when I listen to You, I hear You encouraging me to grow. In Jesus' name, I pray.

Reflection

I'm not a fan of water sports and never really enjoyed aqua aerobics. At the cottage, I prefer to lounge on the dock. But at the gym, my chosen piece of equipment is the Rowing Machine. I choose this because it gives me a total body workout. Also, it's a movement that I can't easily copy at home. Using a treadmill seems redundant given the amount I walk, and I like to bike in the great outdoors.

What's your favourite piece of workout equipment?

Top Tip

Hold your stretch – Stretch all your muscle groups daily and hold each stretch for at least 10 seconds, working up to 30 seconds. Stretching every day is ideal, but at the very least stretch before or after you exercise.

Bible Truth

"God is our refuge and strength, an ever-present help in trouble" (Psalm 46:1 NIV).

Challenge

Express your personal feelings about God in a journal.

Praise Move: Triceps Stretch

Stand, feet shoulder width apart.

Place one hand on the back, between the shoulder blades.

Gently push down on the elbow with the other hand.

Hold and repeat for other arm.

The Sinner's Prayer

The Sinner's Prayer; I never liked the title of this prayer. I had difficulty admitting that I had done wrong, let alone that I was a sinner. I acted nice to my neighbours, friendly to my co-workers. I didn't murder. I led an upstanding life. Yeah, sure I might have told a little white lie or thought something nasty about a person I didn't like, but that doesn't make me a sinner. Or does it?

God doesn't use a scale to measure one sin against another. In His eyes, the fact that I might be envious of a rich person's mansion is as bad as when I stole a pair of earrings as a child. The fact that I might have lustful thoughts for a movie star is as bad as when I lied to my mom about smoking in her car. All of these sins are considered equal.

This is similar to a law in the health field that a calorie is a calorie is a calorie. 3500 calories equals one pound, no matter how we consume the calories. It's a law in nature.

So is the law of sin. A murder is no worse in God's eyes than stealing. In our society, we measure sin on a scale and we strive to find a punishment to fit the crime. This is our legal system. However, I'm not talking about human law but rather the way in which God views sin.

This realization that a sin is a sin is a sin can seem harsh. The fact is that we are all stained with a sinful nature and our sin keeps us from heaven. However, God doesn't leave us here. God gave us His only son to die on the cross in our place for our past sins and our future sins. This gives us reason to rejoice. Although we are sinners in God's eyes, He has made a way for us to be clean and to enter into heaven. All we need to do is say and believe the Sinner's Prayer:

"Lord Jesus Christ, I am sorry for the things I have done wrong in my life. Please forgive me. I now turn from everything that I know is wrong. Thank You that You died on the cross for me so that I could be forgiven and set free. Thank You that You offer me forgiveness and the gift of Your Spirit. I now receive that gift. Please come into my life by Your Holy Spirit to be with me forever. Thank You, Lord Jesus. Amen."

If you say and believe this prayer you can rest on the hope of salvation and God's promise of redemption.

Exercise Your Funny Bone

Stop, drop and roll does not work in Hell.

You Asked

Q: Is my weight on a scale a good indicator of my overall health?

A: Your weight is the sum total of your bones, organs, fat, muscles and other tissue. But body composition (fat compared to lean body mass) is more important. Two people can weigh exactly the same on a scale and yet be tremendously different in body composition. Since muscle weighs more than fat, the scale weight can be deceiving. Instead, pay attention to how you feel and how your clothes fit.

Faith Lift

Dear Lord – I pray that You will grant me the strength and desire to become a better person and be with me as I try to change. In Jesus' name, I pray.

Reflection

Today, my family had plans away from home. Left to work in solitude I didn't leave my desk all day. Although I had a productive day, I realized at the end that I didn't even venture outdoors for a refresher. My fingers got a good workout at the keyboard, but that was about it.

Do you ever get caught up in work and forget about your health?

Top Tip

Team up with a friend – A partner can make workouts more fun and push you to try harder. You'll be more likely to stick to your plan if you have a partner. Join a walking club, a sports team or an aerobics class.

Bible Truth

"Dear friend, I pray that you may enjoy good health and that all may go well with you, even as your soul is getting along well" (3 John 2 NIV).

Challenge

Memorize one new Bible verse.

Praise Move: Back - One Arm Bent-over Row

Bend at the waist and place one hand on a bench so that your back is parallel to the floor and your head is in line with your spine.

Hold a dumbbell in one hand with your arm hanging down directly in line with your shoulder, palm-facing inward, and elbow relaxed.

Slowly pull the weight to the side of your body by flexing the elbow.

Pause and then lower slowly to the starting position. Repeat 10 times.

Repeat for other arm.

Tips:

1. Concentrate on pulling with your back muscles, not your biceps.
2. Keep your back flat and don't rotate your hips or shoulders.
3. Keep one hand on the bench at all times.

Obedience, Not Experience

I'd never led a prayer meeting before – let alone in my bathing suit. However, God doesn't want my experience but rather He wants my obedience. At a women's conference, I learned what this truly meant. The coordinator asked me to lead the morning swim and prayer. Generally, I only use my pool at home to play in with the kids. I'd never been an aqua aerobics leader. I'd only ever attended one water aerobics class. I definitely didn't have the experience. But God didn't ask me for experience, He only wanted my obedience. And when I responded, "Yes, I'll do it" He honoured my obedience.

That morning, I prayed before the class even started. I felt no anxiety as the Holy Spirit guided me in what to do. I started with a quiet prayer, "What would You like me to start with Lord?" and He would provide me with an idea. I would share this with the group and we would do it. Then I'd ask, "What do I do now?" and He would give me another idea. We did this for 45 minutes.

After the swim, I joined the ladies in the locker room and they encouraged me with their comments. God had given each woman what she needed that morning and He used me to do it.

I had learned a motto at a small business seminar over ten years ago that I still live by today, "Get the deal, then panic." The instructor referred to business deals. He advised us to say yes to any request clients or customers brought forward and then later worry about the details. I adopted that motto for my business and enjoyed some very interesting experiences because of it.

However, there is one significant difference between, "get the deal, then panic" and "obedience, not experience" – it's the panic. I know that when God asks me to do something, He will also equip me to do it. There's no need for panic. God will not ask me to do anything for which I'm not ready. I can move forward and say "yes" trusting that I'll have the help I need.

In business, I'm a sole proprietor. In faith, I'm a partner. And what a partner I have. I know that whatever God asks me to do, He will honour my obedience and help me to do it.

Is there anything God is asking you to do that you have said "no" to because you lack experience?

"If they obey and serve Him, they will spend the rest of their days in prosperity and their years in contentment" (Job 36:11 NIV).

Exercise Your Funny Bone

A clock that is stopped is right twice a day.

You Asked

Q: Could I use an electronic stimulation device instead of doing exercises?

A: The amount of electricity needed to stimulate a muscular contraction equal to doing one sit-up would inflict more pain than anyone could tolerate. No device develops a better body without any work on your part. There is no substitute for your own effort.

Faith Lift

Dear Lord – I pray that You will give me extra strength to get through today and every day when I am under pressure. In Jesus' name, I pray.

Reflection

I've learned that if I don't start my day with God, then my day isn't as satisfying as it can be. Without God, I can easily lose the desire to take care of myself. I can return to old habits. In one day, without God's help, I can let go of healthy eating and my desire to exercise.

What impact has inviting God into your life every day had?

Top Tip

Look the part – Put on workout clothes; don't just change into running shoes. If you look the part, you'll feel the part. Keep workout clothes in the car or beside the front door. Wear light, comfortable, non-restrictive clothing, and shoes with a good arch support. Avoid jewelry and wear a safety strap with glasses.

Bible Truth

"I pray that out of His glorious riches He may strengthen you with power through His Spirit in your inner being" (Ephesians 3:16 NIV).

Challenge

Put down your fork between each bite at mealtime.

Praise Move: Shoulder - Standing Overhead Press

Stand with your feet shoulder-width apart.

Hold a dumbbell with an overhand grip at each shoulder, elbows bent at your sides.

Press the weights up slightly in front of you until your arms are completely extended overhead, without locking your elbows.

After a slight pause at the top of the movement, return to the starting position. Repeat 10 times.

Tips:

1. Be careful not to overarch your back.
2. Concentrate on keeping your body stable and abdominals contracted.
3. Don't rest the weight at the bottom of the movement.

Progress, not Perfection

My girlfriend is a runner. She runs every day and even participates in races. She didn't start running until her mid-twenties and she eagerly learned as much about it as she could. She joined a runner's club, hired me as her personal trainer, and bought books on the subject. One day, she shared with me her excitement upon finding a gem of a motivational statement in one of the books. It read, "Strive for progress not perfection."

As a beginning runner, she easily became discouraged watching others win the race when she struggled to finish it. It disheartened her to suffer from shin splints and leg pain after the first few outings. But this became her mantra, "progress, not perfection." She wanted to improve and work toward perfection. However, every day she only needed to see that she had progressed. Each day she had to try.

In our faith journey God expects the same. He doesn't desire perfection, although this is our end goal. He wants to see progress. He wants to see us trying every day to live a Christian life modeled after Jesus. However, some days we may feel discouraged because other people seem more "Christian" than us. Maybe they can memorize and quote scripture or maybe they have a melodic ability to pray. We can feel disheartened seeing others leading people to Jesus when we are still working on ourselves. However, God sees our hearts. He knows our intentions. And although we may fall short of where we'd like to be, God is patient and He wants us to get up, dust ourselves off and continue our walk.

"I have fought the good fight, I have finished the race, I have kept the faith" (2 Timothy 4:7 NIV).

Exercise Your Funny Bone

CH _ _ CH

What's missing? U R!

You Asked

Q: My friend said that sauna suits, plastic wraps and rubber jumpsuits are great ways to lose weight. Is this true?

A: These suits are usually made of a material that holds in body heat, causing perspiration. The perspiring leads to dehydration and a temporary body-water weight loss, not a fat loss. Overheating is not only useless but also dangerous. There is simply no short cut to weight loss.

Faith Lift

Dear God – I pray that when I am weak You will strengthen me and when I lose hope You will increase my faith. In Jesus' name, I pray.

Reflection

I'm feeling good about myself since I started this partnership with God. I have more control over my eating, as I'm more mindful and call on God's strength every day. I feel energized to work in my gardens, continue my daily walks and strength train at least once a week. My clothes feel looser around the waist, so I know I'm losing inches. I think it would be better for me to throw out the scale altogether and rely on how my clothes fit and my energy level as better indicators of my health.

What indicators of health can you rely on instead of the scale?

Top Tip

Vary your routine – You may be less likely to get bored or injured if you change your routine. For example, walk one day and bicycle the next.

Bible Truth

"Finally, be strong in the Lord and in his mighty power" (Ephesians 6:10 NIV).

Challenge

Try working out in small chunks of 10 minutes, three times a day.

Praise Move: Triceps - Overhead Extension

Stand holding a dumbbell in one hand with your arm extended above your head.

Hold your arm vertical, close to your head and without changing elbow position, slowly lower the weight behind your head as far as comfortably possible.

After a pause, slowly lift to the overhead position. Repeat 10 times.

Repeat for other arm.

Tips:

1. Support your vertical arm with your other hand, just below the elbow.
2. Keep shoulder blades down and together throughout the movement.
3. Don't jerk or bounce the weight from the bottom position.

Sabbath

I celebrated a belated honeymoon with my husband. We stayed in a gorgeous hotel that featured a wood burning fireplace and therapeutic tub. It offered the perfect opportunity to put up my feet and relax.

One evening, after a fine meal, we returned to the hotel and noticed a computer sitting alone in the hotel lobby. I felt drawn to this machine. I wanted to check my e-mail. Imagine that. I had five days to be away from my email, cell phone and computer obligations, yet I felt compelled to sit behind the keyboard and check in on work.

How ridiculous. We live in a world driven by technology. Yet instead of giving us more freedom, it seems to have shackled us further.

In the Bible, we are directed to take a day off. A day where we leave the worries of the week and focus our physical and mental energies on God. Now this is something we should be doing daily, but most of us don't take even an hour out of our day to focus on God. We are commanded to take a day off. Silly, really, that we must be told to take time off? We must be reminded to relax?

The Ten Commandments express God's unchanging standards for moral living. In Exodus 20, we are told to, "Remember the Sabbath day by keeping it holy. Six days you shall labor and do all your work, but the seventh day is a Sabbath to the Lord your God." We know that Jesus is the new covenant because He fulfilled the law, but He still wants us to follow the spirit of the law.

After my vacation, I returned refreshed and rejuvenated. I tackled my regular routine with renewed vigour and enthusiasm. Imagine if I did this once a week. Imagine how much better I would feel on Mondays if I only did what God asked of me.

"Observe the Sabbath day by keeping it holy, as the Lord your God has commanded you. Six days you shall labor and do all your work, but the seventh day is a Sabbath to the Lord your God" (Deuteronomy 5:12-14 NIV).

Exercise Your Funny Bone

From a church bulletin: The sermon this morning: "Jesus Walks on the Water." The sermon tonight: "Searching for Jesus."

You Asked

Q: Is muscle soreness a sign of a good workout?

A: Exercise is not supposed to hurt. While a little soreness is normal after you start exercising, pain isn't. The best relief for muscle soreness is rest, and the best prevention is to be careful not to overdo it in the first place.

Faith Lift

Dear Lord – I pray that You draw me closer to You as my strength and comfort. In Jesus' name, I pray.

Reflection

My husband and I took advantage of a holiday and planned a fun outing together -- rollerblading! Our city offers a wonderful paved trail so we left early to beat the crowds. My husband strapped on his blades and patiently waited for me to fasten my helmet, wrist protection, elbow pads and kneepads. Then off we went. Well, off my husband went...I sort of padded along. By the time I had made it to the first resting bench, my shins burned and my legs ached. Never had I experienced such pain in my outer thighs. Forty minutes later, I collapsed in the front seat of our truck. What a ride. I thanked my husband for being a good sport, and suggested we make rollerblading a more frequent activity.

What new sports/activities can you do with your significant other or friend?

Top Tip

Make fitness a family activity – Plan a weekend hike, sign up for line-dancing together, coach your child's sports team, go ice-skating at the local community centre, plan a canoeing vacation, take an after-dinner walk, sign up for a mother-and-child exercise class, or go sledding together.

Bible Truth

"Everything that lives and moves will be food for you. Just as I gave you the green plants, I now give you everything" (Genesis 9:3 NIV).

Challenge

Say a daily prayer of thanks for your health.

Praise Move: Calf Stretch

Stand; take a step forward with one leg.

Bend the front knee while keeping the back knee straight, both feet flat on the floor.

Gently press your body forward and push on back heel of the straight leg.

Hold and repeat for other leg.

Pesky Problems

Today I started out on my walk, breathing in the sweet smell of early morning blossoms. I drank in the beauty of the majestic blue spruce trees reaching to the perfect sky. I eavesdropped on the call of one Blue Jay to another. A truly glorious morning.

Ready to start my time in prayer, I began with thanks to God for the beauty all around me. But then it started; the buzz of a horsefly as it flew near my ear. And again. It circled my head as I walked. I tried to swat it away, but it moved too fast. I pulled the collar of my shirt up over my head so that only the eye of my sunglasses showed. I must've looked like quite the sight. Unfortunately, this strategy not only didn't work, it seemed to excite the pesky fly and I think he called for his friends. Three horseflies surrounded me now.

I returned my shirt to normal and began swatting again. It didn't work. I started to run, thinking I could get away. This didn't deter them. Aha, I thought of using my arms in helicopter motion, alternating my swings so that the fly never had any open opportunity for them to land on my head. I succeeded in hitting them, but I think it actually encouraged them to try harder. I fought in a losing battle.

Funny thing, by this time I walked a third of the way through the neighbourhood and I hadn't even started my prayers. I focused on the problem of these horseflies. I had ignored my Lord in favour of focusing on my problems. When I realized this I straightened my shirt and held my head up high with my arms naturally swinging by my side. I decided to ignore the horseflies and focus on God. I began my prayers.

By the time I had rounded the last corner to my home, the flies had lifted and I walked without aggravation. Coincidence?

There are many times in my life when instead of focusing on God, I pay attention to the problem at hand. I put so much energy into fixing my situation that I ignore my Lord altogether. But God wants to be part of the solution. He wants me to spend my energies on Him.

When I set out on my walk tomorrow, I plan to start with an open heart and a clear focus on my Lord.

Exercise Your Funny Bone

If you're headed in the wrong direction, God allows U-turns.

You Asked

Q: If women lift weights will they bulk up?

A: Women have less of the hormone needed to build muscle bulk easily. Very large muscles are most likely not in their genetic potential. Generally, women can't develop huge muscles without spending hours a day lifting very heavy weights.

Faith Lift

Dear God – I pray that when I make promises to myself and You about all the things I'm going to do, You will help me to follow through. In Jesus' name, I pray.

Reflection

When I go for my morning walk, I'm energized for the day and have clearer thinking. When I lift weights, I'm stronger, not only physically but also in my attitude. I feel good when I awake in the morning. I'm not giving up anything in order to be healthy but instead I feel like I've gained a better quality of life.

What small changes have you made that make you feel better?

Top Tip

Have fun – Take the "work" out of workouts. Try something new and experiment until you find one that you like doing. The best fitness plan is one that you can easily include in your busy schedule and not another thing to add to your "to-do" list. Give thought to activities you enjoyed as a child, a teenager and as an adult.

Bible Truth

"The LORD is my strength and song, And He has become my salvation; This is my God, and I will praise Him; My father's God, and I will extol Him" (Exodus 15:2 NIV).

Challenge

Drink 8 large glasses of water each day.

Praise Move: Biceps - Concentration Curl

Sit on the edge of a bench with your feet firmly on the floor about shoulder-width apart, toes pointed slightly outward.

Keep your back straight, lean forward, and place your left hand on your left thigh just above the knee for support.

Pick up a dumbbell with your right hand, palm facing away from you, and brace the upper part of your right arm against the inside of your right thigh to isolate the biceps.

Curl the weight up toward your right shoulder smoothly.

After a brief pause at the top of the movement, lower the weight with control as you inhale. Repeat 10 times.

Tips:

1. Never throw the weight up or use jerky motions to lift the weight.
2. Use only your biceps and work through the full range of motion.
3. Do the curl with one arm at a time to concentrate on the movement.

Sun Shower

The trail beckoned me to explore it. It had a floor of stone and wood chips and measured wide enough for a small vehicle. I had an hour to myself so I laced my running shoes and started on my walk.

I enjoyed the gorgeous scenery all around. Trees overhanging created a canopy of green and yellow. Streams of water flowed under an old wooden bridge. Blue jays and chickadees called to each other. The wind tossed poplar leaves that made a sound like rushing water. I hoped to spot a moose, but prayed not to see a bear. Unfortunately (and fortunately) I didn't see either. I had hit the 30-minute mark and with no end in sight, I decided to turn around.

Descending a small hill, I felt a few drops of rain. Looking up to the sky, a big black cloud loomed over me. The drops turned into a spray and the spray quickly changed to a shower. I pulled my hooded sweater over my head and walked closer to the edge of the trail to steal shelter from the trees.

I whispered a prayer to God, "Lord, will You stop this rain until I get home?" His response to me? "No, but I will give you this," and with that a burst of sunshine came through the clouds. A sun shower. I smiled.

God reminded me that there are times in life when we're in a situation that we don't like and although we want God to rescue us, He may choose to let us experience the pain for reasons we may never understand. He may not pull us out of the trouble or stop the ugliness altogether, but God will never leave us. He will always be with us through it. He is like the sun in a sun shower.

"We are hard pressed on every side, but not crushed; perplexed, but not in despair; persecuted, but not abandoned; struck down, but not destroyed" (2 Corinthians 4:8-9 NIV).

Exercise Your Funny Bone

From a church bulletin: Our youth basketball team is back in action Wednesday at 8 PM in the recreation hall. Come out and watch us kill Christ the King.

You Asked

Q: If I exercise a lot do I need to have extra protein in my diet?

A: Most people get more than enough protein in their diet. The average person, even if she exercises a lot, doesn't need a high-protein powder, drink, tablet, capsule or bar. Feeding your body more protein than it needs won't help. Excess protein is converted to energy and then burned up or stored as fat.

Faith Lift

Dear Lord – I pray that You pump up my energy when I feel exhausted and my spirits are low. In Jesus' name, I pray.

Reflection

Yesterday, my doctor's appointment took over two hours. This left little time to prepare a meal, let alone do my strength training. However, instead of "throwing in the towel" and giving up entirely, I chose to reschedule my weight lifting session and grabbed a semi-nutritious meal. I experienced a wonderful change to my usual knee jerk reaction.

When things don't go as planned, and time is robbed from you, what may you do instead?

Top Tip

Follow your program – Strength train two to three times per week, every other day. Leave 48 hours rest in between your workouts. For example, strength train on Monday, Wednesday and Friday or Tuesday, Thursday and Saturday. Don't work the same muscles on consecutive days.

Bible Truth

"The thief comes only to steal and kill and destroy; I have come that they may have life, and have it to the full" (John 10:10 NIV).

Challenge

Call a friend to go out for a walk together.

Praise Move: Quadriceps Stretch (front thigh)

Stand, with one hand on a wall for support, hold ankle of outside leg.

Gently press foot down into hand.

Never pull foot up towards buttocks.

Hold and repeat for other leg.

Water Sports

I blame my experiences as a child on my dislike of water sports today. I remember three specific events that lead me to be a land-lover. The first happened when, as a pre-teen, my dad took me water-skiing. A pretty good sport, I even enjoyed jumping the wake from the boat. But then I fell. The fall itself didn't hurt and I didn't injure myself. But I landed in a bed of seaweed and could feel the slippery tentacles crawling up my legs and clawing at my life jacket. It was all I could do not to scream in terror. My father turned the boat around and when he pulled me in, I vowed never to water-ski again.

The next summer, I sat as a passenger in a speedboat with a maniac driver. He thought it fun to scare children by going as fast as he could and making the boat wobble. The terror seized me so badly that I had to seek a place to hide under the bow of the boat. I vowed never to go in a speedboat again.

Lastly, as a teenager, I agreed to go fishing with two friends in a canoe. We were staying at a remote hunting lodge. Leaving early in the morning, we paddled to the end of a marshy lake before the middle passenger decided to stand and move around. Our canoe flipped over, spilling all the contents, including us, into the frigid spring waters. We managed to pull the canoe to shore. Soaked, cold and scared, we loaded ourselves back in, without our gear, and returned to the camp. I vowed never to go in a canoe again.

Fast forward to today. My husband and children are camping in a park in Quebec. My husband wakes me up in the early morning hours, excited to invite us all on a 5-hour trek to a remote waterfall. I grudgingly enquire about this voyage, and then quickly decline his invitation when I find out that half of the trip is by canoe. "No way." My husband counters with claims that it'll be the "best fun ever" and I would regret it always if I didn't join the family. In the back of my mind, I'm reminded that God didn't give me a spirit of fear but one of power. With this scripture in mind, and the coaxing of my husband, I agree to go.

I write this now, in the safety of my office, with a grin on my face. I will never forget that trip. Laurentian Mountains towered over our canoe. A majestic waterfall met us at the end of a one-hour hike uphill. At the falls, we ate sandwiches and the kids splashed in the waters. We returned to our campsite, although a little worn out, a happy family.

My husband knew me best; I would have regretted not going. I'm grateful that the Lord reminded me that fear is not from Him. If I let fear rule my day, I would have missed out on one of the best experiences of my life.

"For God did not give us a spirit of timidity, but a spirit of power, of love and of self-discipline" (2 Timothy 1:7 NIV).

Exercise Your Funny Bone

From a church bulletin: Ladies, don't forget the rummage sale. It's a chance to get rid of those things not worth keeping around the house. Don't forget your husbands.

You Asked

Q: I don't have much room in my apartment. Do I need specialized equipment to weight train?

A: Ordinary floor exercises that work with the body's own weight can give an excellent and complete muscle workout. Weights and other specialized equipment are great for isolating muscles and for working against high resistance. However, you don't need specialized equipment to build muscle fitness.

Faith Lift

Dear God – I pray that You will guide me through my goals and help me to stay committed without the guilt. In Jesus' name, I pray.

Reflection

It felt good to move my body as I did as a child. Today, I played Frisbee, kicked the soccer ball around and had a wonderful after-dinner bike ride with my family. Fitness isn't about doing aerobics and going to the gym. It's about enjoying the quality of your life and getting out there and moving.

What physical activities did you enjoy as a child?

Top Tip

Select your exercises – It's important to have an overall development of the body and perform strength training exercises in the order of larger muscle groups to smaller ones: legs, chest, back, shoulders, arms, and abdomen.

Bible Truth

"Love the Lord your God with all your heart and with all your soul and with all your mind and with all your strength" (Mark 12:30 NIV).

Challenge

Create an exercise area to call your own.

Praise Move: Hips Stretch

Stand, step forward with one leg – take as long a stride as possible.

Bend knee and drop back leg until you feel gentle tension in the front of the hip.

Hold and repeat for other leg.

First Impressions

"Are you familiar with the saying, 'You never get a second chance to make a good first impression'"? Working for years as an Employment Counselor, this question stood out as one of my favourite lines to share with clients during our interview workshops. But what does it mean to make a good first impression?

As a gift, a friend gave me a book called, "Dress Your Best – The Complete Guide to Finding the Style That's Right for Your Body". Whatever your body type, this book tells you what to wear to make yourself look your best. One of the premises of the book is not to be dissatisfied and try to change how you look, but instead to make yourself look your best today.

The better you look today the more you'll be motivated to be healthy. I've found that as I mature and grow in my Christian walk I can find new freedom. God created me to be beautiful. I don't need to worry excessively over my appearance. One friend shared, "Where before I wanted to be the centre of attention so I took to preening before I would put my head out of the door, now I am happy in the skin of who I am in Christ and no longer need that attention. Not to say I want to look….slovenly. But, I don't mind running to town in my track suit without makeup. I like the fact that people look at me deeper inside and not the outside. It is extremely liberating. I have more friends now who know the "real me"."

Appearance is more than how I look. How I feel also feeds into this first impression. God is changing my appearance; both how I look and how I feel. How about you?

Exercise Your Funny Bone

From a church bulletin: Remember in prayer the many who are sick of our community. Smile at someone who is hard to love. Say "Hell" to someone who doesn't care much about you.

You Asked

Q: Can I "spot reduce"(lose weight from specific areas of my body) by exercising the muscles there?

A: No diet or program is going to take the fat off of any particular area of your body. You can reduce overall body fat, but you can't selectively take fat off a specific area of your body.

Faith Lift

Dear Lord – When I look in the mirror, I pray that You will help me be gentle with the person I see. In Jesus' name, I pray.

Reflection

With summer here, my schedule is no longer my own. My routine has run amuck and I must cater to my children first. As far as exercise goes, I get it where I can. I join my son for a game of badminton in our backyard. I work my leg muscles with a weight-training workout with a girlfriend as our children play together. I bike around the block with my daughter. I walk with my husband as the sun sets in the evening. It's not the same routine, but I am still keeping active living as a priority.

How can you keep your activity level up?

Top Tip

Move slowly – Concentrate and isolate the muscles that are being exercised. Raise and lower the weights under control and don't let momentum take over. Moving slowly is best as too much momentum takes resistance off working muscles.

Bible Truth

"Do not be anxious about anything, but in everything, by prayer and petition, with thanksgiving, present your requests to God. And the peace of God, which transcends all understanding, will guard your hearts and your minds in Christ Jesus" (Philippians 4:6 NIV).

Challenge

Take the stairs whenever possible.

Praise Move: Chest Stretch

Stand, bring arms behind back.

Clasp hands together and gently pull arms back and up.

Hold.

Need to Pump Iron

Chronic fatigue started to get me down. I'd go to sleep as early as my children and have difficulty getting out of bed twelve hours later. I'd then have to nap later in the afternoon. Upon my husband's insistence, I finally made a doctor's appointment.

My doctor ordered a series of tests, most of which I couldn't even pronounce. Three weeks later, the results are in. I am iron deficient. I thank God that I wasn't diagnosed with a life threatening disease. Iron deficiency is something that can be easily managed.

Iron is an essential mineral for life. It's found in red blood cells and its job is to carry oxygen from the lungs to the rest of the body. This oxygen releases energy from the foods you eat. Some characteristics of low iron include weakness, lethargy, muscle fatigue, and shortness of breath. My doctor recommended iron supplement pills and choosing more colourful foods such as red meats, dark green vegetables and the browns of whole grains.

Looking into it further, I learned that iron from meats, the "heme" form, is more easily absorbed than that from vegetables. In general, meat, fish, and poultry are excellent sources. Organ meats like liver, kidney and heart are important sources. Others include beets, egg yolks, legumes, kale, sardines, oysters, anchovies, mussels, and clams. This will call for a revamping of my diet. Some food sources that I have in my kitchen right now include raisins, dried apricots, spinach, broccoli, beans, dried fruits, whole grains, fortified cereals, and enriched breads.

Unfortunately, one friend told me that caffeine could inhibit the body's absorption of iron. In researching this, I found out that indeed tea and coffee contain inhibitors. To my surprise, my desire to increase fiber in my diet may also have worked against iron absorption. According to a pamphlet published by the Beef Information Centre, "A high fiber intake in general may act as an iron inhibitor." They recommend eating foods that contain heme iron and /or vitamin C when eating foods that act as iron inhibitors. For example, eating a spinach salad that has strawberries is a good combination; beans with tomato sauce and pork; spaghetti with meat sauce; a glass of orange juice with a bowl of oatmeal cereal. God truly blessed us with many food options. With summer here, I can easily make these ideas part of my weekly diet. I'm ready to start "pumping iron".

Exercise Your Funny Bone

From a church bulletin: For those of you who have children and don't know it, we have a nursery downstairs.

You Asked

Q: Will walking with weights on my wrists or ankles burn more calories?

A: Walking with ankle weights can increase risk of injury to your hips, knees, ankles and feet. Wrist weights can cause shoulder and elbow injuries. This adds stress to the body in a way that it wasn't designed to handle, and the increased calorie burn is negligible.

Faith Lift

Dear Lord – I pray that You will assist me in making the plans I need to get started and to stay on track. In Jesus' name, I pray.

Reflection

I really shouldn't leave the decision to exercise up to whether I feel like it or not. As the Nike ad says, I need to "just do it". When I think about whether I really want to spend time on the rowing machine and whether I really want to press 300 lbs. then I can easily talk myself out of it. Next week, I'm going to buy that gym membership and commit to go, no matter how I feel.

What slogan motivates you?

Top Tip

Cool down and stretch – After your workout, repeat part of your warm up and stretching routine to help your muscles recover. Remember to drink lots of water.

Bible Truth

"I can do everything through Him who gives me strength" (Philippians 4:13 NIV).

Challenge

Buy a good pair of walking shoes.

Praise Move: Neck Stretch

Stand, feet shoulder width apart.

Turn the head as if to look over one shoulder.

Hold and repeat for other side.

Fasting

When I attended high school I participated in a 30-hour fast with a group of fellow students. It felt like the longest hours of my life! I felt faint and nauseated and had trouble thinking of anything but food. It reminded me of times when I would try silly diets like eating only cabbage soup or grapefruits at every meal. It seemed the harder I tried to fast the more I focused on what I didn't have.

When church friends invited me to fast as an adult, I quickly rejected the notion. I didn't want to feel sick and deprived. I didn't want to think about food all the time. However, with this new invitation came some direction and guidance that opened my eyes and my heart to the true meaning of fasting.

First of all, I learned that I could fast in many different ways. I could abstain from all food and liquids, except water; or I could skip all food but drink liquids like juice, broth and herbal tea; or I could give up certain foods. I learned that fasting is not so much about going without something as it is about using the time I would spend on that activity to pray.

I learned that fasting acts as a reminder to pray. Every time I felt hungry, I would be reminded to pray. Fasting is a time to abstain from the physical and devote my attention to God.

There are many mentions of fasting and prayer in the Bible. I learned that people fasted for a number of different reasons including during times of celebration, in petitioning God for healing, for His intervention for victory in battle, and in preparation for ministry. In the Old Testament, Ezra 8:23 says, "So we fasted and petitioned our God about this, and He answered our prayer." Nehemiah 1:4 says, "When I heard these things, I sat down and wept. For some days I mourned and fasted and prayed before the God of heaven."

In the New Testament, Jesus began His ministry with prayer and fasting. And the first missionary journey began with prayer and fasting.

Many of us can't physically go away to a quiet place to pray yet we can pray as we go about our daily routine. We can begin our day fasting and then pray while driving, walking or cooking. I plan to spend time in prayer asking God how He would like me to participate in a fast. How about you?

"So after they had fasted and prayed, they placed their hands on them and sent them off" (Acts 13:3 NIV).

Exercise Your Funny Bone

From a church bulletin: The Fasting & Prayer Conference includes meals.

You Asked

Q: Should I continue working out even if I hurt myself?

A: You can still workout after any injury if you modify your workout to exercise around the injury. For example, if you hurt your ankle, it wouldn't be a good idea to jog on it, but you may still be able to do other light exercises in a pool.

Faith Lift

Dear God – I pray that You instill in me a responsibility to care for my body, to nourish and sustain it. In Jesus' name, I pray.

Reflection

Yesterday afternoon, I looked around my home. The amount of housework that had piled up over the course of the week daunted me. I felt overwhelmed so decided to first take a power nap. I prayed that when I awoke I'd have the energy to tackle the work. Not only did I awake feeling energized but also I worked on projects that I hadn't even planned.

God answers prayers both big and small. What are you in need of today?

Top Tip

Know the terms – "Free weights" are bars with weight plates on each end. A "barbell" is a long bar and a "dumbbell" is a short bar. A "bench" is usually a flat support similar to a piano bench. An "ankle weight" is a weight that can be wrapped around your lower leg. "Repetitions" (reps) means completing a performance of a single exercise, which includes both up and down. A "set" is the number of repetitions of a given exercise.

Bible Truth

"So do not fear, for I am with you; do not be dismayed, for I am your God. I will strengthen you and help you; I will uphold you with my righteous right hand" (Isaiah 41:10 NIV).

Challenge

Schedule exercise into your daily planner…in ink!

Praise Move: Hamstrings Stretch (back thigh)

Stand; take a small step forward with left leg.

Raise left toes, keep heel on floor, knee straight.

Lean forward with straight back.

Hold and repeat for other leg.

Fanatical

1991 – Laurier faced Mt. Allison at the Sky Dome for the Vanier Cup. Six of my girlfriends and I decided to go to the championship football game.

We drove from Waterloo to Toronto, and then took the subway into downtown. The excitement in the air energized me. Most fans dressed in the WLU colours of purple and gold. I remember wearing a gold coloured scarf to support my team.

Once at the stadium, we found our seats and joined in the cheering. What a game! I had never been to a football game and so my best friend described to me exactly what happened. Caught up in the brouhaha I yelled and screamed until my throat felt raw. I'm not sure why I even bought a seat because I didn't sit down for the entire game. I waved my scarf up in the air until my arms were tired. You can imagine the burst of sheer joy when my team won the cup. The party continued late into the night. Elated that my team had won and proud to be a Laurier student I strutted around happy to be on the winning team.

Remembering that football game reminded me of a poster my son had in his bedroom. It pictured a muscle-clad man sporting a t-shirt with the motto, "Be on the winning team!" At the bottom it clarified, "God's team."

I am a member of God's team. I joined when I gave my heart to Jesus. I feel proud to be a Christian. I am happy knowing that when I die I'll go to heaven.

Funny though, one would think that my salvation is a little more important than my favourite team winning a sports event. Knowing where I'll spend eternity is a tad bit more inspiring than a plaque on the wall with the year of the championship. Why don't I treat it as such?

Why can I go to a football game and scream, jump and raise my arms in support of my team, yet on Sundays at church, I am reluctant to even raise a hand? Why is it that as a fan of a sporting event I feel it's okay to act fanatical, but within the walls of my own church family I'm much more reserved?

This year, I resolve to act more enthusiastic about what truly matters in life. I'm going to sing out loud, cheer, and yes, I'm going to raise both my arms at church.

"David, wearing a linen ephod, danced before the LORD with all his might, while he and the entire house of Israel brought up the ark of the LORD with shouts and the sound of trumpets" (2 Samuel 6:14-15 NIV).

Exercise Your Funny Bone

Does your life stink? Do we have a pew for you!

You Asked

Q: Should I work out hard during a cold or flu?

A: Your body tries to fight illness and if you overtax it with strenuous exercise you could run the risk of getting sicker. Once you're better, use shorter, less intense sessions to build slowly back up to your former level.

Faith Lift

Dear Lord – I pray that when temptations cross my path, You will give me the strength to resist. In Jesus' name, I pray.

Reflection

Today, I decided to reward myself for achieving my goals so far. It's important to notice my accomplishments as I go along instead of reaching a goal and then looking forward to the next goal. While it's motivating to have goals to work towards, I realize the importance of celebrating the ones I've attained. Then I'm not always living in the future and anticipating things to be better "then". I can enjoy now, look back to see where I've come from, celebrate my successes, and continue to be motivated to move on.

How can you take the time to notice your accomplishments?

Top Tip

Celebrate goals reached – Every time you reach a goal, celebrate. Reward ideas may include making a long-distance phone call, treating yourself to a long bubble bath, getting a pedicure, facial or massage, buying an extravagant bouquet, or subscribing to an exercise magazine.

Bible Truth

"God saw all that He had made, and it was very good" (Genesis 1:31 NIV).

Challenge

Pack a bag for all your workout needs.

Praise Move: Abdominals - Basic Crunch

Lie on your back on the floor, your knees lifted directly above your hips, legs hip-width apart and your calves parallel to the floor.

Place your hands behind your head, fingertips touching.

Contract your abdominals and lift your head, neck and shoulders off the floor as one unit. Feel your abdominals contract or tighten as your shoulder blades clear the floor.

Repeat 10 times.

Tips:

1. Maintain a fist's-width distance between your chin and chest.
2. As you do the crunch, don't hold your breath.
3. Briefly hold the crunch as the top of the lift before returning to starting position.

Tis the Season

Unfortunately, colds can hit us in any season. I've experienced some of the worst summer colds, worse than some of my winter ones. There is no cure for a cold but there are some things I do to help my body fight off viruses: exercise regularly, drink plenty of fluids and eat chicken soup, and stay home in bed to rest.

We all know the importance of exercise. But did you know that the payoff for long-term, regular exercise is lifelong immunity? Research has found that the immune systems of elderly women who were active walkers were as robust as those of women in their 20s. I learned that I can't catch a cold or the flu by getting wet or chilled, so I try to get outside for my exercise.

Other ways I enhance my immune system include taking small amounts of vitamin C regularly, drinking water, eating yogurt, garlic, fruits and vegetables, and washing my hands often with soap and warm water.

My favourite way to keep sickness at bay is to get sufficient sleep. In the deepest phase of sleep, the pituitary gland increases its production of the growth hormone, which in turn stimulates the gland that is at the root of the immune system. Generally, I tend to resist rest because I have so much to get done. But, trying to do more on less sleep is counterproductive. Did you know that we are five times more likely to catch a cold or flu when we try to run on less hours sleep because we are stressed?

A friend had this to share about getting enough sleep: "Yes, rest, so that our bodies, those wonderful and intricate creations of God have down time in order for all of the complex systems to replenish their energy and function as He intended. Like every gift God has given us, we should cherish our health and nourish our bodies."

From being active every day to choosing foods carefully to getting enough sleep, simple lifestyle changes can help your body optimize your immunity.

Exercise Your Funny Bone

From a church bulletin: The peacemaking meeting scheduled for today has been canceled due to a conflict.

You Asked

Q: My friend exercises two times a day, 7 days a week. Is she exercising too much?

A: If you exercise too much your body will hold onto its main resource of fuel, which is fat. Also, exercising too much compromises your immune system and increases your risk of injury. Take at least one full day to recover with little or no activity. The body needs a day of rest, especially if you are starting out.

Faith Lift

Dear God – I pray that I can trust You to be with me always as a loving, sustaining and supporting Presence. In Jesus' name, I pray.

Reflection

Sometimes to clean the bathrooms, grocery shop, prepare meals and take kids to soccer takes priority over exercise. Household chores can get the best of me and by the time I remember to workout, I am lying in bed ready for sleep. The lesson? I must schedule it into my day. I must literally write it on my calendar. Time is a precious commodity and I want to spend mine wisely. The dirty dishes will still be there tomorrow, but I can't say the same for my health.

How can you make exercise a priority in your day?

Top Tip

Choose a weight – Select a strength training weight that is heavy enough so that it's tough to complete the last few reps of each set but not so tough that form and technique are compromised. Follow this rule of thumb: if you can only do six reps, then decrease the weight, and if you can do 12 reps easily, then increase the weight. Be sure to work on better technique and higher reps before adding any weight to your exercises.

Bible Truth

"Jesus looked at them and said, 'With man this is impossible, but with God all things are possible'" (Matthew 19:26 NIV).

Challenge

Go to bed 30 minutes earlier than normal every evening for a week.

Praise Move: Buttocks Stretch

Sit with right leg lying forward along the floor.

Left leg is bent at the knee, foot on the floor across the outstretched leg.

Right hand pulls the bent knee into the chest and turn head behind the back.

Hold and repeat for other leg.

Care for the Caregiver

I settled in for a long plane ride from Canada to Europe to attend my brother's wedding. The flight attendant instructed us on seatbelt use, emergency exits, and oxygen masks. She reminded us of the importance of taking care of our own needs first, before helping the person next to us – whether a small child, elderly parent, or someone struggling with their mask. The explanation seemed simple. We are no good to anyone else if we don't take care of our needs first…if we pass out before we get our own mask on, we won't be able to help the person next to us.

This philosophy can be applied to all areas of our life. Unfortunately, many of us don't heed this simple logic. We tend to put the needs of others over and above our own. We care for children first, then our spouse or significant other takes priority, followed by work obligations and maybe even volunteer work, and we inevitably put our own needs last. We think that at the end of the day, if we are not already exhausted, we may then spend some time on ourselves.

However, it's important to fuel the body, mind and spirit on a daily basis through proper eating, relaxation techniques, prayer, and exercise.

We need to fuel our bodies with adequate foods and not skip a meal because "we don't have time." Food gives us energy.

Also, realize that pampering ourselves with a warm bath, practicing stretches or taking time to read from a favourite book should not send us spiraling into the depths of guilt.

Prayer, when combined with quiet time, can decrease respiratory rate, heart rate, elevated blood pressure and muscle tension. During prayer, the body escapes from the stresses of everyday life and enters into a relaxed state.

Finally, keep in mind that energy begets energy. If we're feeling tired and rundown, that's the time that we really need to focus on increasing our exercise. A brisk walk or strength-training program can give us the boost we need to motor through the day. Remember, when we feel nourished and energized, we are better able to deal with all the demands in life. Taking time for you is not selfish; it's necessary!

Exercise Your Funny Bone

From a church bulletin: The Rector will preach his farewell message after which the choir will sing "Break Forth Into Joy."

You Asked

Q: Does it matter what kind of shoes I wear for aerobics?

A: The shoe should match the sport. Walking shoes are designed for forward movement, and they don't offer a lot of side-to-side support for an activity such as aerobics. Use comfortable footwear that provides good cushioning and support.

Faith Lift

Dear Lord – I pray that You help me to feel Your love and strength every day, and that with You beside me, I can endure all things. In Jesus' name, I pray.

Reflection

Autumn is upon us and with the cooler weather I find myself searching in my closet for warmer clothes. I don't like the idea of adding bulk to my frame, but layering is the best way to go at this time of year. With cooler mornings and higher temperatures in the afternoon, it's a good idea to wear outfits that can be shed as the day goes on.

Have you kept your wardrobe equipped to match the weather?

Top Tip

Change the routine – Vary strength training exercises and equipment using a combination of free weights, machines and tubing. There are a variety of ways to increase the intensity of a given workout. One is by adding more weight. Another method of increasing the intensity is to decrease the amount of time required to complete a given workout.

Bible Truth

"She sets about her work vigorously; her arms are strong for her tasks" (Proverbs 31:17 NIV).

Challenge

Stretch every day upon waking while saying, "This is the day the Lord has made. Let us be glad and rejoice in it!"

Praise Move: Back Stretch

On all fours, curve the back upwards.

Keep head turned down.

Hold.

Goals and Rewards

Goal planning is one of my favourite activities. I would like nothing more than to sit down with pen in hand and a desk-size calendar to map out my goals. This is one of the reasons I loved working as a personal trainer; I delighted in creating health plans for my clients.

What are the benefits of setting goals? Goals give you the direction, energy and purpose you need to get going. Goals decrease stress and give you a sense of control and accomplishment.

Goals need to be specific. A vague goal is unlikely to be accomplished. First, a complex or long-term goal needs to be broken down into smaller or shorter-term goals to ensure success. Then, the way to know whether you have accomplished your goal is if you have some way to measure it. Ideally, you can use numbers to track your progress and achievement. Thirdly, to ensure success, make your goal is attainable and achievable. Lastly, without a realistic deadline it's too easy to procrastinate. A time limit will help you stay focused on your goal.

To say, "I want to lose weight" is not specific enough. To say, "I want to lose 100 pounds in three weeks" lacks realism. Instead, a more specific and realistic goal starts, "I will lose 10 pounds in two months." Or "I will lose two inches from my thighs in three months." Or "I will cycle three miles to the grocery store by the end of the month." You get the idea.

If you've always used food as your reward this will not be effective especially when you're trying to change your eating lifestyle. If you find that there's really nothing you don't give yourself whenever you want it, try taking the emphasis off of buying something. Instead revamp your reward system to include reading a book or magazine for fun, watching an old movie or doing activities you haven't done in a while just for fun, like playing 4-square or catch-the-flag.

Exercise Your Funny Bone

From a church bulletin: A bean supper will be held on Tuesday evening in the church hall. Music will follow.

You Asked

Q: I heard it's not a good idea to start strength training until I am within 25 pounds of my ideal weight. Is this true?

A: Strength training is a cornerstone of weight management. By lifting weights, you build muscle. This extra muscle boosts metabolism, making you burn more calories even when at rest and thereby helping you to lose fat and keep it off.

Faith Lift

Dear Father – I pray that when I reach out and open my heart, You will be there as my source of strength, comfort and love. In Jesus' name, I pray.

Reflection

I noticed I needed a larger social circle to help me stay on the right health and fitness track. It's easy to lose balance and lose control. Friends and family help me to remain focused.

What have you done to build and maintain a circle of people to support you?

Top Tip

Start in position – Begin your strength training and stretching program from a comfortable position, such as standing or lying on the floor. If your balance is poor, start by doing some activities on a chair, on your bed or supported by a wall.

Bible Truth

"I love You, O LORD, my strength" (Psalm 18:1 NIV).

Challenge

Replace your mid-afternoon coffee break with a tall glass of water and piece of fruit.

Praise Move: Shoulder Stretch

Stand, arm behind back.

Hold wrist with other hand.

Bend elbow and gently pull your arm across your back.

Hold and repeat for other arm.

Pause for Menopause

I once shared an office with a woman who experienced symptoms of menopause. At times she felt so warm that she needed to take off layers of clothing and fan herself. Although I'm years away from menopause, it's a natural phase in life and something I can plan for now.

During menopause, a woman's estrogen production decreases as her ovaries cease to function. It is possible for a woman to lose as much as 30% of her bone mass during this period, leading to postmenopausal osteoporosis. Also, risk for developing heart disease increases after menopause. In addition to physical changes, the signs of menopause may include mood swings, depression, irritability and anxiety.

But there is something women can do. Women who have participated in lifelong physical activity typically have a higher bone mineral density at the start of menopause than inactive sedentary women do, and so have an advantage. Exercise lowers blood pressure and raises the level of good cholesterol, protecting the heart. Exercise does other good things for women after menopause. It strengthens the endocrine system so that the adrenal glands and ovaries function more efficiently. It helps women lose weight, taking some stress off the heart, joints and all other body systems. Physical activity helps to relieve stress, anxiety and tension. It's been proven to increase energy levels and promote deep, restful sleep. We know that it increases our sense of mental well-being. It can make women feel stronger, more self-assured, and even look better.

My personal favourite exercise is brisk walking, but low impact aerobics, rowing, jogging and dancing are all "weight-bearing" activities that help keep bones strong. Also effective are "resistance" exercises such as weight training.

By improving circulation, exercise can make a menopausal women's body more tolerant of temperature extremes that hot flashes bring on, and I can reap all the above benefits as well.

Exercise Your Funny Bone

From a church bulletin: Potluck supper Sunday at 5:00 PM - Prayer and medication to follow.

You Asked

Q: I want a flat stomach. Should I do sit-ups every day to exercise my stomach?

A: The abdominals should be treated the same way as other muscle groups and so they don't need to be exercised every day. Doing a lot of crunches won't slim your waist. The best way to lose fat is with cardiovascular and strength training exercises.

Faith Lift

Dear God – I pray that when I give my heart to You, I will experience joy and inner peace on a daily basis. In Jesus' name, I pray.

Reflection

Yesterday, I stopped my chores and laced my running shoes in preparation for a weight lifting session. Although my body felt weak, my spirit was willing. I turned on Christian music and sang along as I went through my exercises. In the end, I felt more energized. Instead of wasting time coming up with excuses of why I didn't want to do it, I committed my energy to completing the program.

Like loud music, what else could you put into place to motivate you to move your body?

Top Tip

Watch your technique – Don't bounce or force a stretch. Use gentle, smooth movements. Gradually ease into it and stretch to where you feel a slight, mild tension, never to the point of pain.

Bible Truth

"I praise you because I am fearfully and wonderfully made; your works are wonderful, I know that full well" (Psalm 139:14 NIV).

Challenge

Take 5 minutes each day to sit quietly and listen.

Praise Move: Biceps Stretch

Stand beside a wall, place one hand behind the back onto the wall.

Without moving the feet, turn the shoulders away from the wall.

Hold and repeat for other arm.

Mirror, Mirror

How easy (or difficult) is it for you to stand in front of a mirror and say, "I'm beautiful"?

Don't feel like trying? Tried it, but have trouble believing it? Remember that God's Word, the Bible, tells you that He created you. He loves you and He wants you to love yourself. You are beautiful. He has made everything beautiful. (Ecclesiastes 3:11) It's extremely important for you to feel good about yourself, no matter what your size, or looks, or ability. God wants you to be the most beautiful and useful person you can be. Your value is not found in physical appearance but in being a child of God.

Don't just endure life, enjoy it! You can enjoy healthy living – physically and spiritually. Taking care of your body and tending to your spirit adds joy to your life.

A friend of mine shared, "As for believing I am beautiful, well, God has been working with me on that one for the past year. Today, I can actually tell myself (and believe it on most days) that I am as God made me – beautiful, loving, gracious, strong, healthy, and of sound mind. I thought the exact opposite of this for most of my life. It is amazing how believing God's words and denying Satan's attacks can actually change how we see ourselves. It has been a slow process. However, positive talk does work to change our worldly beliefs."

Remember, God loves beauty and He created you.

Exercise Your Funny Bone

From a church bulletin: Next Thursday there will be tryouts for the choir. They need all the help they can get.

You Asked

Q: Is it true that I will lose flexibility as I age?

A: Flexibility is specific to the individual, the activity, and to each joint. The more frequently and regularly you stretch, the more flexible you'll remain as you age.

Faith Lift

Dear God – I pray that as today is a new day, help me to be a new person in You. In Jesus' name, I pray.

Reflection

Sometimes I don't feel motivated to do my strength training program, but I've done three things to make it more appealing: 1) I've designed a program that can be completed in 30 minutes, 2) I've set up a mini-weight room in my basement, and 3) I play my favourite Christian music.

How can you make your exercise activities more appealing?

Top Tip

Remember to breathe – Don't hold your breath when exercising or stretching. When stretching, breathe in a natural rhythm – inhale deeply and then exhale slowly.

Bible Truth

"It is God who arms me with strength and makes my way perfect" (2 Samuel 22:33 NIV).

Challenge

Each morning, look in the mirror and say, "I am God's daughter. He loves me!"

Praise Move: Abdominals Stretch

Lie on your back; straighten out your arms and legs.

Point fingers and toes to stretch as far as you can.

Hold.

CONCLUSION

I started my health and fitness journey by writing in a journal. Over the course of the following weeks, I improved my health – physically and spiritually. I pray that this devotional has set you on a course to improve your health through the seasons as well.

Blessings as you continue on your journey to improved spiritual and physical health!

About the author

Kimberley Payne is a motivational speaker and writer. Her writing relates raising a family, pursuing a healthy lifestyle and everyday experiences to building a relationship with God. Kimberley offers practical, guilt-free tips on improving spiritual and physical health. Visit her website www.kimberleypayne.com

*

Did you enjoy this book? Please take a moment to write a review. Share the blessings.

A little star review will do!

Other Books by Kimberley Payne

Fit for Faith – 7 weeks to improved spiritual and physical health
Want to get on the road to a healthy body and spirit? Discover ways to balance the physical and spiritual.

Get the Skinny – Answers to 45 Frequently Asked Health & Fitness Questions
Have health, weight and fitness questions? Learn the answers to live healthier and happier lives.

JumpStart – A Catalyst to Launch you into a Daily Spiritual & Physical Health Routine
Want to make simple changes to improve spiritual and physical health? Discover a daily, specific program to create a routine.

Healthy Body, Healthy Spirit: 4 Key Habits to Improve Your Personal Health
Want to learn from the experts? Discover these four key habits to set your life.